PILL POTENCY:

A Pharmacist's Guide to Vitamins and Supplements

By

Andy M. Johnson

TABLE OF CONTENTS

INTRODUCTION

Pill potency refers to the strength or effectiveness of a medication contained within a pill or tablet. It indicates the concentration of the active ingredient(s) in the medication, which is responsible for producing the desired therapeutic effects. Understanding pill potency is crucial for both healthcare professionals and patients, as it directly influences the dosing and efficacy of a medication.

Pill potency is typically expressed in terms of the amount of active ingredient present per unit of the pill, often measured in milligrams (mg) or micrograms (mcg). The potency of the medication can vary widely depending on factors such as the drug's chemical composition, manufacturing process, and intended therapeutic use.

For healthcare providers, accurate knowledge of pill potency is essential for prescribing the appropriate dosage to achieve the desired therapeutic effect while minimizing the risk of adverse effects. Pharmacists play a vital role in ensuring that the dispensed medications match the prescribed potency, promoting patient safety and treatment effectiveness.

Patients, on the other hand, should be aware of the potency of the pills they are prescribed or are taking over the counter. Understanding pill potency helps patients follow their healthcare provider's instructions regarding dosing frequency and quantity, which contributes to the medication's optimal effectiveness and overall well-being.

It's important to note that variations in pill potency can occur due to factors such as differences between generic and brand-name medications, changes in manufacturing processes, and storage conditions. Therefore, maintaining open communication with healthcare professionals and pharmacists is crucial to ensure that patients receive the intended potency of their prescribed medications.

CHAPTER 1

INTRODUCTION TO DIETARY SUPPLEMENT

A manufactured substance known as a dietary supplement can be taken as a pill, capsule, tablet, powder, or liquid to complement your diet. To boost the amount of nutrients consumed, a supplement can include either synthetic or nutrients that have been derived from dietary sources. Vitamins, minerals, fibre, fatty acids, and amino acids are among the group of nutritional molecules. Additionally, dietary supplements may contain ingredients like plant pigments or polyphones that are touted as having positive biological effects but have not been proven to be necessary for survival. Ingredients for supplements can also come from animals, such as fish or chicken collagen. These can be blended with nutritious substances and are also sold alone and in sets. Additionally, the European Commission has set uniform guidelines to ensure that dietary supplements are secure and properly labelled.

Dietary supplements are goods that can be consumed with meals or at certain intervals to complement a person's daily diet and are meant to improve their health and wellness. When a vitamin is deficient or there is an imbalance, supplements are necessary. As of 2013, the global market for nutrition and supplements was worth over US$104 billion. Demand for mineral supplements is rising due to an ageing population, a rise in the number of pregnant women, and an increase in urbanisation. Due to excessive dietary supplement usage brought on by the increased demand, consumers may be exposed to health risks. Vitamins, minerals, proteins, multivitamins, multi-minerals, herbs, carbs, hormone activators, and oil supplements are some of the several categories of dietary supplements.

Dietary supplements are widely utilised and fall under a large group of ingestible goods that can be distinguished from everyday foods and medications. In the US, dietary supplements are products that contain at least one of the following ingredients: vitamin, mineral, herb, or botanical (including extracts of herbs or botanicals), amino acid, metabolite, or any combination thereof. These products must not be tobacco products. In brief, nutritional supplements include items like multivitamins, garlic tablets, fish oil capsules, probiotics, organic weight-loss aids, and particular kinds of energy drinks.

Dietary supplements, whether they come in the form of tablets, capsules, powders, or liquids, must be identified as such on their labels and be exclusively meant for oral administration. Additionally, unless the chemical component has previously been sold as a dietary supplement or food, dietary supplements may not contain chemical compounds that have been licenced as biologics or pharmaceuticals. In retail settings, supplements are frequently offered alongside traditional over-the-counter drugs. Many customers frequently see dietary supplements as alternatives to traditional drugs, even though they are not meant to treat, cure, alleviate, or prevent any disease.

CHAPTER 2

WEIGHT LOSS SUPPLEMENT

It's tempting to look for assistance everywhere when you want to lose weight. When considering dietary supplements or herbal therapies, keep in mind that many of them have received mixed ratings from research. The claims aren't always well supported by evidence, and some might pose health hazards. Before attempting any, first, speak with your doctor.

You should also be aware that the FDA has taken action against several weight reduction products that contained prescription medicines but failed todisclose this on the label. Sometimes it's impossible to know what you're getting.

The FDA does not regulate supplements the same way it does food and medications. Before these supplements hit the market, the FDA does not examine them for efficacy or safety.

Chitosan

This particular sugar is derived from the tough skin of lobsters, crabs and prawns. It can allegedly prevent your body from absorbing fats and cholesterol.

Does it aid in weight loss? According to Natural Medicines, a non-profit organisation that reviews the research on dietary supplements, there isn't enough trustworthy evidence to assess it. Chitosan has not been proven to be beneficial for assisting with weight loss, according to the National Centre for Complementary and Integrative Health.

Although chitosan often has minimal adverse effects, some persons experience constipation or an upset stomach. Chitosan should not be taken if you have a shellfish allergy because it is a product of shellfish.

Chromium Picolinate

The mineral chromium improves the hormone insulin, which is crucial for converting food into energy. It is also necessary for your body to store proteins, lipids, and carbohydrates. There are claims that chromium supplements can:

- Lower your appetite
- Help you burn more calories
- Cut your body fat

- Boost your muscle mass

However, a study of 24 research that examined the effects of chromium intakes ranging from 200 to 1,000 mcg per day revealed no appreciable advantages. Chromium is "possibly ineffective" for weight loss, according to Natural Medicines.

Chromium supplements are normally safe for people at doses lower than 35 mcg per day. Higher doses may result in:

- Insomnia
- Irritability
- Problems thinking
- Headache

Additionally, ingesting chromium has caused kidney damage in some people. If you have kidney issues, you should avoid using it.

Conjugated Linoleic Acid (CLA)

This is a well-known supplement that contains substances present in linoleic acid, a fatty acid. There are claims that it could support weight loss efforts and keep you satisfied.

The evidence on CLA's role in weight loss is conflicting. According to some, taking 1.8 to 6.8 grammes of CLA per day may:

- Curb body fat
- Build muscle

However, according to some studies, it doesn't aid in weight loss.

According to Natural Medicines, CLA is "possibly effective" for reducing weight.

Long-term use, particularly if you're obese, may increase insulin resistance, which increases your risk of developing type 2 diabetes, according to some researchers. Additionally, it may drop "good" cholesterol in your blood, increasing the risk of heart issues.

CLA side effects in some persons could include:

- Upset stomach
- Nausea
- Loose stools
- Fatigue

Glucomannan

It is produced using the Konjac plant. Similar to other dietary fibres, it is intended to aid in weight loss by preventing the absorption of fat from food into the body.

Early research suggests it might be beneficial, while other data indicate it is ineffective.

According to Natural Medicines, there is "insufficient evidence" to determine the effectiveness of glucomannan for weight loss.

If you take glucomannan in the supplement's tablet form, you run the risk of choking or developing a blockage in your:

- Throat
- Esophagus (the tube that connects the throat to the stomach)
- Intestine

If you take this supplement as a powder or a capsule, it seems to be a little bit safer.

Additionally, glucomannan might hinder your body's ability to absorb drugs. So either take your medication an hour before or four hours after using glucomannan.

Green Tea Extract

It supposedly works by:

- Curbing your appetite
- Raising calorie and fat metabolism

According to Natural Medicines, there isn't enough data to assess how effectively it functions.

When used in large doses, green tea extract can have the following negative effects:

- Nausea
- Vomiting
- Bloating
- Gas
- Diarrhoea
- Dizziness
- Insomnia
- Agitation

Green Coffee Extract

Early study indicates it might result in a minor decrease in weight, but more trials are required. According to Natural Medicines, there isn't enough high-quality research to determine whether it is effective. Few people experience negative effects, however, because green coffee contains caffeine, they could include:

- Headaches
- Stomach upset
- Nervousness
- Insomnia
- Abnormal heart rhythms
- Gas
- Diarrhoea

Hoodia

This particular plant can be found in Africa's Kalahari Desert. The National Centre for Complementary and Alternative Medicine states that Bushmen historically utilised the stem of the root to quench their thirst and quench their hunger during protracted hunts. Currently, it is promoted as an appetite suppressor.

P57, a component included in hoodia, is thought to reduce appetite by making you feel satiated. However, there is no solid proof that it is secure or efficient. Natural Medicines claims that there is insufficient data to determine the efficacy of hoodia.

7-Keto-DHEA

Your body naturally contains this. By increasing your metabolism and causing you to burn more calories throughout the day, it might aid in weight loss.

In a few short studies, those who took 7-keto-DHEA lost considerably more weight than those who received a placebo (a fake pill). This was in conjunction with moderate activity and a low-calorie diet. Natural Medicines, however, claim that there is yet insufficient solid information to assess how effectively it functions.

Ephedra

This herb is also referred to as ma huang. From a closely related species that grows in North America, this plant is distinct. Ephedrine, a stimulant, is present in ephedra.

It is very closely connected to these artificial substances that are present in some drugs:

- Pseudoephedrine
- Phenylpropanolamine

The FDA outlawed ephedra-containing products because the herb was connected to major adverse effects, such as:

- Heart attack
- Arrhythmia
- Stroke
- Psychosis
- Seizures
- Death

Traditional Chinese herbal medicines and items like herbal teas are exempt from the FDA's restriction. The FDA states that the herb's benefits are largely limited to temporary weight loss. The organisation claims that any benefits outweigh the health hazards. Ephedra, according to Natural Medicines, is "likely unsafe."

Bitter Orange

Africa and tropical Asia are the native home of the bitter orange tree. Additionally, it is grown in Florida, California, and the Mediterranean. Synephrine, a stimulant linked to ephedrine, is found in the bitter orange fruit peel. It allegedly functions by increasing the amount of calories expended.

Many manufacturers switched to bitter orange after the FDA outlawed weight reduction pills containing ephedra, but it's unclear if it's safer.

According to Natural Medicines, bitter orange is "possibly unsafe" when taken orally as a supplement, and there is insufficient proof to determine whether it aids in weight loss.

According to certain research, taking supplements containing bitter oranges can increase your heart rate and blood pressure. According to reports, those who consumed bitter oranges either alone or in combination with other stimulants like coffee may have had harmful side effects. The dangers comprise:

- Stroke
- Irregular heartbeat
- Heart attack
- Death

According to the FDA, using bitter oranges as a dietary supplement may not be safe. If you suffer from a heart issue, high blood pressure, or another illness, you ought to stay away from it in particular.

If you take coffee, some drugs (like MAO inhibitors), herbs, or other supplements that raise the heart rate, you should also stay away from bitter orange supplements.

CHAPTER 3

HEART HEALTHY SUPPLEMENTS

Your bones, muscles, and many other body parts can benefit from supplements. How is your heart? According to research, some of them may assist with blood pressure, cholesterol, and other factors that increase your risk of heart disease. However, it's uncertain whether they aid in shielding against heart attacks, strokes, and other issues.

These vitamins and minerals might be a beneficial addition to your heart-healthy diet.

Fibre and Sterols for Your Heart

Fibre: Fibre, which is present in foods including fruits, grains, vegetables, and legumes, reduces the amount of cholesterol your body absorbs from food. Try to consume 25 to 30 grammes of it daily. Men who are under 51 years old should aim for 38 grammes per day. The easiest way to acquire your recommended daily intake is through eating, but supplements are also an option. Blond psyllium husk, a frequent ingredient in fibre supplements, has strong scientific support for its ability to reduce "bad" LDL cholesterol. It can also increase HDL, the "good" sort. Methylcellulose, wheat dextrin, and calcium polycarbophil are further dietary fibre supplements. If you use a fibre supplement, gradually increase your intake. By doing this, cramps and gas can be avoided. Additionally, it's critical to consume adequate water when upping your fibre consumption. **Both stanols and sterols**: These can be obtained as supplements or found in foods like nuts and cereals. They lessen the quantity of cholesterol that is absorbed by your body from diet. They are also included in a variety of foods, including yoghurt, various kinds of margarine, and orange juice. For those with excessive cholesterol, experts advise 2 grammes per day to help decrease LDL cholesterol.

Additional Supplements That Could Be Beneficial

Coenzyme Q10 (CoQ10): This enzyme, also known as ubiquinone and ubiquinol, is produced in minute quantities by your body regularly. Taking CoQ10 as a supplement, either by itself or in conjunction with drugs, may help decrease blood pressure.

As a remedy for the negative effects of cholesterol-lowering medications known as statins, CoQ10 supplements are also widely used. Why? Sometimes, these medications can reduce the amount of CoQ10 that the body naturally produces. In an effort to make up for the loss, some doctors advise taking a CoQ10 supplement in the hopes that it may help with issues like muscle discomfort and weakness. However, the body of scientific research does not generally support the use of CoQ10 for muscle soreness brought on by statins.

Magnesium: Magnesium can occasionally be used to assist repair irregular heartbeats in addition to maintaining normal blood pressure.

Rice with red yeast: Several studies suggest that red yeast rice may reduce "bad" LDL cholesterol, triglycerides, and total cholesterol. Monacolin K, a component of red yeast rice, is the same as the active component in medication for lowering cholesterol. Before consuming red yeast rice, see your doctor.

Use of Safe Supplements

Never use a supplement simply because it bears the phrase "heart healthy." You can acquire too much of some of them, and not all of them are certain to be helpful to you.

Consult your doctor to learn the safe maximum limits and suggested daily amounts for the vitamins you take. Make sure you need the supplement by paying close attention to what it accomplishes. Which product is most likely to be helpful? Ask your doctor. You must heed your doctor's recommendations if you have a heart ailment or are at a high risk of having a heart attack. Attempting to cure a major medical issue on your own with over-the-counter supplements is far too dangerous.

Fatty fish: It is rich in omega-3 fatty acids and can reduce blood levels of triglycerides, an unhealthy fat, by up to 30%. Furthermore, it might lower blood pressure. However, there is no proof that omega-3 fatty acids reduce your chance of developing heart disease. Eating fish rich in omega-3 fatty acids can be your best option. All people should have two servings of fish that are 3.5 ounces or less per week, according to the American Heart Association.

Garlic: It not only enhances the flavour of almost everything but may also modestly lower blood pressure. It might lessen your risk of blood clots by slowing the development of plaque in your arteries. According to research, garlic in diet and supplements may be beneficial.

Herbal tea: According to research, both the extract and the beverage may increase HDL levels and lower LDL and triglyceride levels.

Linseed oil: It's possible that flaxseed and flaxseed oil decrease cholesterol. It's unclear if it also reduces your overall chance of developing heart disease.

Acid folic: The B vitamin folic acid reduces homocysteine levels, which has been related to heart disease. However, research has not demonstrated that folic acid lowers the frequency of subsequent heart attacks and strokes.

Supplements that may be good for your heart

Four supplements stand out among the many others that promise to boost heart health in terms of the amount of research available.

Omega-3 fatty acids, start Omega-3 fatty acids might lessen the body's inflammatory response, which might lessen some risk factors for heart disease.

It has been demonstrated that omega-3 fatty acids slightly reduce blood pressure. They may also lower triglyceride levels, as well as inflammation and plaque accumulation in the arteries, which may minimise the risk of a heart attack. It has also been demonstrated that omega-3 fatty acids (found in fish oil) lower the risk of sudden cardiac mortality brought on by erratic heartbeats.

Omega-3 fatty acids can be obtained in sufficient amounts from foods like fatty fish like salmon or trout as well as from plant sources like walnuts and flaxseed. High triglyceride levels can also be treated using FDA-approved prescription drugs that include omega-3 fatty acids, such as Lovaza and Vascepa.

B9 vitamin folate

Vitamin B9, often known as folate, is a crucial water-soluble vitamin. Some individuals may be at an increased risk of stroke if they have low levels of folate and high amounts of the amino acid homocysteine. Homocysteine may erode artery inside walls. The breakdown of homocysteine by folate in the body lowers the risk of stroke and cardiovascular disease, according to high-quality research. Supplemental folate has been demonstrated to be helpful for persons with low folate levels who do not already have heart disease. The effects of folate on other populations, including those with pre-existing cardiac disease and those with normal folate levels, require additional study.

Vitamin D.

Low vitamin D levels raise the risk of heart attack, stroke, and hypertension in individuals. Blood pressure was reported to drop after taking vitamin D supplements, but only in people with high blood pressure and vitamin D insufficiency. In those with high blood pressure but normal vitamin D levels, vitamin D did not lower blood pressure.

If you are already taking any medications, make sure to see your healthcare professional before taking vitamin D supplements. Some heart drugs that can also elevate calcium levels may interact with vitamin D's ability to enhance calcium levels in the body. Digoxin, diltiazem, verapamil, and hydrochlorothiazide are a few of these.

Magnesium

It has been discovered that taking oral magnesium supplements can lower blood pressure in those who are on blood pressure medication. Magnesium, however, has not been proven to significantly lower blood pressure in persons whose blood pressure is already under control.

Which supplements are unlikely to help your heart health?

Here are four supplements that are frequently promoted as having positive effects on heart health but whose usage is not well-supported by research.

1. B6 vitamin

Some claim that a slight vitamin B6 deficiency can raise the chance of developing cardiovascular disease. Some people think that taking vitamin B6 will reduce their chance of developing heart disease because this vitamin is necessary to reduce homocysteine.

Overall, nevertheless, the claim that vitamin B6 lowers the risk of heart attack is unsupported by the available research. Furthermore, there is little evidence that vitamin B6 lowers the incidence of stroke.

The majority of adults and kids get enough vitamin B6 each day through foods including fruit, starchy vegetables, and animal products. Additionally, even though your body will absorb vitamin B6 from supplements, a significant amount of it will pass through urine.

2. Coenzyme Q10

The body naturally produces coenzyme Q10 (CoQ10), which is present in the heart, liver, and other organs. There are instances when persons with heart disease have reduced levels of CoQ10. People have therefore hypothesised that supplements may lower your risk of developing heart disease.

Coenzyme Q10 may help reduce cardiovascular risk factors such as high blood pressure, high cholesterol, and blood sugar balance, according to certain small studies. Additionally, coenzyme Q10 might lower the possibility of various problems following cardiac surgery. There isn't much proof, though, that it combats heart disease. Any advantages for heart health require further study to be confirmed.

3. Antioxidants

Antioxidants are known to lessen oxidative stress, a condition in which molecules damage cells and can result in several illnesses. Antioxidant supplements are known to lower the risk of cancer and heart disease. Antioxidants as supplements are not advised for heart disease prevention, despite evidence that oxidative stress can affect heart health. Instead, eating more fresh produce that is high in antioxidants, such as fruits and vegetables, may help lower the risk of heart disease.

4. Each day's multivitamin

Multivitamins do not significantly reduce the chance of developing heart disease. It is not necessary to take a daily multivitamin if you eat a balanced diet.

If you eat too many fat-soluble vitamins, your body may store them and they may cause more harm than benefit.

Dietary Supplements That May Be Harmful To Your Heart

Many supplements contain natural substances, yet there may still be hazards associated with using them. These dietary supplements could be dangerous.

• L-arginine: When combined with prescribed blood pressure drugs, L-

arginine may significantly reduce blood pressure and cause bleeding. Additionally, it is risky for those who have experienced a past heart attack.
• Supplements containing garlic: Whether consumed fresh or as pills, garlic can raise your risk of bleeding. If you currently use blood thinners, this may be an even bigger problem.

What then will improve the health of my heart?

Making changes to your food and way of life can help you improve your heart health naturally and effectively.

Reducing salt intake for heart health

Cutting back on sodium intake can help lower your risk of developing high blood pressure and heart disease. You can reduce your dietary salt intake by:

• Restricting your consumption of highly processed foods, such as deli meats, salted pretzels, and chips, which are frequently rich in salt. Fast food and other frozen meal options are examples of convenience foods that frequently have too much salt.

• You may improve the flavour of your food and use less salt by using herbs, spices, and various vinegars while you cook.

• You may make your sauces and dressings using extra virgin olive oil, your preferred herbs, and spices rather than purchasing them. You may regulate the amount of salt and fat in your food in this way.

Changing your diet and lifestyle to improve your heart health

Better heart health is frequently associated with the DASH and

Mediterranean diets. However, any dietary regimen that emphasises plant-based foods, whole grains, healthy fats, and lean protein can support improved heart and general health.

Alcohol, animal products, and added sweets should all be limited if you want to reduce inflammation. Heart disease and other illnesses are connected to chronic inflammation.

You can also alter your way of life to promote heart health by:

- Regular exercise
- Quitting smoking
- Maintaining a healthy weight

In addition to making these lifestyle adjustments, it's critical to schedule routine exams with your doctor. By doing this, you can assist your medical team in assessing your risk and developing a treatment strategy as necessary. If you have a personal or family history of heart disease, this is very crucial.

CHAPTER 4

SUPPLEMENTS FOR BRAIN AND HEALTH COGNITIVE

In addition to being important as you become older, cognitive health is important whenever you want to have more energy, clarity, and attention. While experts concur that a healthy diet and way of life are two crucial elements for brain health, research indicates that some supplements may also be able to promote cognitive and mental health, particularly for older folks, those on limited diets, and those managing particular medical conditions.

Learn which scientifically supported supplements may protect or increase brain function before you start buying and read professional advice on how to maintain mental acuity as you age.

Why Diet is Important for Brain Health

Beyond providing energy for the body and brain during the day, nutrition has an impact on cognitive health. In reality, the nutrients in your diet have an impact on how your brain works and can affect your risk of developing neurodegenerative diseases.

"The brain requires essential nutrients to function properly," says David Seitz, M.D., the medical director of Ascendant, a New York facility for the treatment of drug dependency. "Eating a balanced diet full of fresh produce, whole grains, healthy fats, and complex carbohydrates will assist supply the vitamins, minerals, and antioxidants required for clear thinking and memory recall. Furthermore, he continues, "Adequate nutrition is essential for healthy brain development throughout childhood, adolescence, and even into maturity.

Your brain and mental health can be affected by what you eat or don't consume, adds Lindsay Delk, a registered dietitian and the proprietor of Food and Mood Dietitian in Texas. She points out that the MIND diet was created especially to support brain function and lower the risk of dementia.

The MIND diet incorporates components of the DASH and Mediterranean diets. It concentrates on nutrients like green leafy vegetables, berries, nuts, complete grains, fish, chicken, beans, and olive oil that help improve brain function, according to Delk.

Registered dietician Kristin Gillespie of Virginia Beach suggests that whenever possible, consumers obtain their nutrition from food rather than supplements. "Nutrients found in foods tend to be more readily absorbed by the body compared to the synthetic forms found in supplements," she says. She continues, rather than concentrating on a single nutrient or a small number of nutrients, foods also supply additional nutrients and beneficial chemicals.

Dr Seitz continues by saying that when you get your nutrients through food, you don't have to worry about getting too much or too little, unlike when you take a supplement. However, using supplements to make up for any nutrient deficiencies in your diet might be beneficial. "A supplement may be required for people whose diets may be deficient in these nutrients (i.e., those with absorption issues or who are adhering to restricted diets)," says Gillespie.

The Best Brain Supplements, Per Professionals

Although experts concur that a balanced diet and way of life are the most crucial factors in promoting brain health, research indicates that the supplements listed below can assist fill in significant nutrient gaps in a person's diet—and possibly promote mood and cognitive health.

The fatty acids omega-3

Omega-3 fatty acids top the list of all supplements advised by specialists for maintaining brain health. "Omega-3 fatty acids, particularly the long-chain fatty acids DHA and EPA present in fatty fish, are essential for the development of the brain and the eyes and have a significant influence on mental health at all ages," observes Eva De Angelis, a licenced dietitian nutritionist and chef based in Argentina.

According to Delk, these fatty acids contribute to the reduction of inflammation in the body and the brain and are linked to a lower risk of dementia, Alzheimer's disease, and cognitive decline.

EPA and DHA levels are typically lower in persons with neurodegenerative illnesses, and omega-3s play critical roles in the membranes of nerve cells. Omega-3s may also help protect against neurodegeneration and lower the risk of cognitive decline, according to a study. For all individuals, a daily dose of 1.1 to 1.6 grammes of omega-3 fatty acids is advised. About 1,000 milligrammes (or 1 gramme) of fish oil, including about 300 milligrammes of omega-3s specifically, are present in a normal fish oil supplement. Before selecting a supplement, carefully read the product labels as dosage varies considerably.

Creatine

Creatine supplements are frequently used to increase muscle mass and athletic performance, but a recent study indicates creatine may also help with brain function.

Creatine may help people recover from concussions and minor traumatic brain injuries, reduce the symptoms of depression, enhance cognition, and help guard against neurodegenerative illnesses, according to a 2022 review of the data published in the journal Nutrients. In one study cited in the analysis, adding creatine to the diet benefited older persons' memory.

A naturally occurring amino acid, creatine can be found in the brain and muscle tissue. It is crucial for generating energy, particularly when there is an increase in metabolic demand, such as when one is sleep deprived.

The Internal Society of Sports Nutrition (ISSN) states that healthy people can safely consume up to 30 grammes of creatine monohydrate per day for five years. The ISSN advises starting with a daily dose of around 0.3 grammes of creatine per kilogramme of body weight (for instance, 20 grammes of creatine for a person weighing 150 pounds) for five to seven days, then moving up to 3 to 5 grammes per day after that. It's crucial to follow the dosage guidelines because consuming too much creatine at once can harm the liver or kidneys. notably when there is an increased metabolic demand, such as when there is a lack of sleep.

Caffeine

Coffee drinkers around the world have long suspected that caffeine enhances cognitive function. According to a 2016 review of the available evidence published in the journal Practical Neurology, caffeine can boost alertness and feelings of well-being, enhance focus and mood, and lessen the symptoms of depression. Even the risk of cognitive decline and Alzheimer's disease is lower as a result.

According to Susan Hewlings Ph.D., vice president of research affairs at Radicle Science, "Caffeine is very popular for cognitive function because it has demonstrated neuroprotective benefits."

Simply don't go overboard. Depending on the brew strength, experts advise limiting caffeine consumption to no more than 400 milligrammes a day and no more than 200 milligrammes at a time. Consuming too much coffee may cause agitation, sleeplessness, and palpitations.

L-Theanine

The amino acid L-theanine occurs naturally in certain mushrooms, green tea, and black tea. According to many studies, it helps with focus and mental function, says registered dietician Leah Johnston of Chicago.

Participants in a brief experiment published in the journal Neuropharmacology made fewer mistakes than those who received a placebo before a monitored two-hour task period[3].
Studies evaluating the effects of L-theanine supplementation on cognitive performance frequently employ daily doses between 100 and 250 milligrammes, even though there is no defined dose recommendation or upper limit. L-theanine concentrations in green tea range from 8 to 30 milligrammes per cup.

Nutrition D

Despite being known as the "sunshine vitamin," vitamin D is essentially a hormone, according to expert dietitian Sascha Landskron of the United Kingdom. She continues, "Vitamin D is crucial for maintaining good brain health and has hundreds of important physiological functions."

According to research, vitamin D is crucial for the early stages of brain development and a lack of it has been related to diseases like dementia, melancholy, autism, and schizophrenia. According to a 2017 study published in Current Gerontology and Geriatrics Research, vitamin D helps elderly persons preserve cognitive function. Although exposure to sunlight is the best source of vitamin D, Landskron warns that you may need a supplement if you work inside, apply sunscreen, cover your skin, have darker skin, are obese, work outdoors in the winter, or if you have darker skin. Cod liver oil, fatty fish like salmon and trout, mushrooms, fortified cereals, and milk are all excellent sources of vitamin D. The recommended vitamin D intake for most persons is between 600 and 800 IU. However, long-term vitamin D supplementation can have negative health effects, such as excessive blood calcium levels that can obstruct blood vessels or result in kidney stones. To establish the ideal dosage of vitamin D supplements for your body's requirements, think about having your vitamin D levels examined and speaking with your doctor.

Choline

Jacques Jospitre, Jr., M.D., a board-certified psychiatrist and co-founder of SohoMD in New York, explains that choline, which is a natural substance found in eggs, is a necessary nutrient that aids in the brain's production of acetylcholine, a neurotransmitter required for memory and general cognition.

People who took large levels of choline seemed to have a lower risk of cognitive deterioration, according to one research of more than 2,000 older adults[5]. Dr Jospitre continues, "More human clinical trials are required, but animal studies show some promise in terms of choline's role in lowering amyloid plaques and Alzheimer's disease risk."

Resveratrol

Resveratrol, an antioxidant polyphenol found in abundance in red wine and grapes, may enhance blood flow to the brain, decrease cognitive decline, and protect cells from injury. Adash Bajaj,

M.D., an expert in anti-ageing and longevity in Los Angeles, says that taking resveratrol supplements could stop the degradation of the hippocampus, a crucial portion of the brain connected with memory.

The National Institutes of Health (NIH) say it's safe to use resveratrol supplements up to 1,500 mg per day for up to three months. Even though higher doses of up to 3,000 milligrammes are safe, they are more likely to irritate your stomach. Because resveratrol can slow blood coagulation, it should be avoided by those who are getting ready for surgery or taking blood thinners.

Mushrooms with a lion's mane

According to Johnston, lion's mane mushrooms (Hericiumerinaceus) provide several health advantages, including lowering inflammation, alleviating anxiety or depression, and boosting cognitive function.

Kara Landau, a prebiotic and gut health expert located in New York, claims that lion's mane mushrooms can improve memory, focus, and concentration by promoting brain oxygen flow. "I find that incorporating [lion's mane mushrooms] daily helps one have a clearer mind and be able to take on the day without the negative side effects of increasing caffeine [intake]," she claims.

To determine your body's tolerance, Landau advises starting with 250 to 500 milligrammes of lion's mane mushrooms every day and working your way up to about 1 gramme. Be aware that lion's mane mushrooms can inhibit the body's ability to coagulate blood, much like resveratrol can. Some people may develop a rash as a result of it.

Vitamin B

The eight B vitamins are crucial for maintaining healthy brain function. According to De Angelis, the vitamin B complex is essential for promoting normal brain function and may guard against memory loss, cognitive deterioration, and neurodegenerative illnesses.

According to De Angelis, particular vitamins B6, B9 (folate), and B12 are required for the metabolism of homocysteine, a chemical produced during the metabolism of methionine. High blood homocysteine levels raise the risk of neurodegeneration and cognitive decline because they can lead to oxidative stress and DNA damage, according to the author.

The majority of people can get all the B vitamins they need by eating a healthy, balanced diet. To meet their needs, a supplement might be necessary for older persons, vegans, and people with specific medical disorders. Adults should consume between 1.2 and 2 milligrammes of vitamin B6, 400 to 600 micrograms of folate, and between 2.4 and 2.8 micrograms of vitamin B12 each day, according to the recommended dietary allowance (RDA). The majority of B vitamins are secure, yet taking too much vitamin B6 can harm your nerves.

Theobromine

According to Landau, theobromine, a naturally occurring stimulant present in chocolate, helps people feel more alert without causing the jittery sensation frequently connected with products containing caffeine. Theobromine may be useful for improving cognitive ability by increasing blood flow to the brain, according to animal and in vitro research, but further human trials are required.

A tasty, abundant source of theobromine, according to Landau, is a daily cup of brewed cacao.

The probiotic and prebiotic

According to Hewlings, gut health is another crucial element for optimum brain performance. The gut-brain axis, which links the gastrointestinal tract and the central nervous system through bidirectional neuronal, hormonal, and immunological signalling pathways, is how probiotics can improve cognition, according to her.

A probiotic combination of Bifidobacterium bifidum BGN4 and

Bifidobacterium longum BORI specifically appeared to enhance brain function and reduce perceived stress in healthy older adults after 12 weeks of supplementation in a 2021 study published in the Journals of Gerontology Series A: Biological Sciences and Medical Sciences. Prebiotics, non-digestible fibres found in cereals, fruits, and vegetables, enhance gut health by feeding good bacteria in the stomach. Galacto-oligosaccharides (GOS), a type of prebiotic, are advised by Landau for supporting both gut health and mood. According to her, the prebiotic GOS has been shown to support mental wellness. Landau suggests that as little as 5.5 grammes of GOS per day may reduce anxiety.

A wide variety of fruits, vegetables, and grains high in prebiotic fibre, as well as fermented foods like kimchi, yoghurt, and sauerkraut that naturally contain probiotic bacteria, can help support healthy gut flora in addition to probiotic and prebiotic supplements.

Magnesium

Although magnesium plays several vital physiological roles, research on how it affects the brain and cognition is still in its early stages. By preventing the deterioration of brain and nervous system cells, magnesium supports appropriate neural function. Numerous studies indicate a link between insufficient magnesium intake and an increased risk of dementia and cognitive decline.

In a 2022 study of more than 2,500 adults aged 60 and older, it was discovered that those who received the most magnesium through diet and supplements performed better on cognitive tests than those who consumed the least magnesium. Low magnesium levels during middle age were linked to an increased risk of dementia but not cognitive impairment, according to another lengthy study. In both studies, it's not obvious if low magnesium levels cause dementia or whether those who already have the disease have low magnesium levels for some other reason.

Numerous plant- and animal-based meals, such as leafy greens like spinach, legumes, nuts, seeds, and whole grains, are rich in magnesium. For adult men and women, the RDA for magnesium is between 310 and 420 milligrammes.

Healthy individuals don't need to be concerned about consuming too much magnesium because the kidneys filter out excess magnesium. But when taken in excess, excessive amounts of magnesium supplements might cause toxicity or gastrointestinal problems including nausea and diarrhoea.

PS, or phosphatidylserine

A group of phospholipids called phosphatidylserine (PS) is naturally present in the membranes of brain tissue. PS influences the release of chemical messengers known as neurotransmitters and activates key signalling pathways, both of which are necessary for communication across the nervous system. According to studies, taking a PS supplement may help safeguard brain health, reduce the risk of developing CNS disorders like

Parkinson's and Alzheimer's disease, and enhance cognitive function by lowering inflammation in the brain.

Phosphatidylserine (PS) supplementation at a dose of 300 milligrammes daily may improve cognitive function and memory without adverse effects, according to a review and meta-analysis published in the Korean Journal of Food Science and Technology in 2022.

However, much of the research that is still in existence on PS is outdated, small, and very briefly conducted.

While further research is required to determine whether PS supplements might enhance brain health and cognition, the preliminary results are encouraging.

PS does not yet have a recommended dose, however, studies indicate that daily doses of 300 to 500 milligrammes are both safe and side-effect-free.

Water

Staying hydrated is one of the simplest strategies to improve brain function. Water makes up around 73% of the brain and central nervous system. According to Dr Jospitre, proper hydration is essential for both the entry of nutrients and the removal of toxins from the brain. "Adequate water consumption may seem obvious, yet most people don't receive enough of it to maintain optimal brain health.

The Institute of Medicine of the National Academies advises adult women to drink about 11 cups of water daily and adult men to drink about 15 cups, including fluid from fruits, vegetables, and other meals that are high in water content.

Even water, though, can be deadly in very large doses. If you consume more water than your kidneys can handle, the sodium levels in your blood can become dangerously low, which could cause psychosis, a coma, and even death.

How to Buy Supplements for Cognitive Health and What to Look for

Dr Jospitreadvises staying away from any supplement that makes a promise about being able to quickly prevent or reverse cognitive loss while selecting ones to support cognitive health. There are no supplements that have been scientifically demonstrated to be able to make these claims on their own, even if additional nutrients are very useful and [may] have research supporting their effects. Every time something seems too good to be true, it generally is, he says.

Before taking any supplement, Landau advisesdetermining how many nutrients are included. She explains that numerous products "add 'fairy dust' amounts of a hyped nutrient to attract consumers but never offer any significant amount associated with clinically proven benefits." On the other hand, certain supplements might contain dosages that are higher than what is advised, which over time could represent a toxicity risk.

Delk suggests buying high-quality supplements from a reliable supplier because supplements aren't subject to the same FDA regulations that medicines are. Choose a supplement that has been put through third-party testing and has the good manufacturing practises (GMP) certification, she advises.

Last but not least, before beginning any new supplement, always speak with a medical expert to be sure it's safe for you and won't conflict with other prescriptions you're already taking.

Salmon Oil

Docosahexaenoic acid (DHA) and eicosapentaenoic acid (EPA), two forms of omega-3 fatty acids, are abundant in fish oil supplements. Numerous health advantages, including increased brain function, have been associated with these fatty acids. Your brain's structure and functionality are crucially maintained by DHA. In actuality, it makes up 90% of the omega-3 fat and about 25% of the total fat in your brain cells. The brain may be shielded from harm and ageing by the anti-inflammatory properties of EPA, the other omega-3 fatty acid in fish oil. In healthy individuals with inadequate DHA intakes, taking DHA supplements has been associated with enhanced thinking, memory, and reaction times. People who are suffering a moderate deterioration in brain function have benefited from it as well. EPA, in contrast to DHA, isn't necessarily associated with enhanced brain function. However, it has been linked to advantages like enhanced mood in depressed individuals. It has been demonstrated that taking fish oil, which containsboth of these fats, can help lessen the deterioration in brain function brought on by ageing. However, there is conflicting information about fish oil's ability to preserve brain health. Overall, eating two meals of oily fish each week is the most effective approach to obtaining the recommended quantity of omega-3 fatty acids. It might be advantageous to take a supplement if you are unable to control this. Numerous supplements are available online.

To determine the optimal amounts and ratios of EPA and DHA, more study is necessary. However, it is typically advised to consume 1 gramme of mixed DHA and EPA daily to preserve brain function.

Resveratrol

Naturally occurring in the skin of purple and red fruits like grapes, raspberries, and blueberries, resveratrol is an antioxidant. Red wine, chocolate, and peanuts also contain it. The hippocampus, a crucial area of the brain connected with memory, may not deteriorate as a result of taking resveratrol supplements. If this is the case, this therapy may help delay the deterioration of brain function that comes with ageing.

Resveratrol has been found to enhance memory and brain function in animal tests as well. One study also discovered that consuming 200 mg of resveratrol every day for 26 weeks improved memory in a small group of healthy older adults. There isn't enough human research done right now, though, to be certain of resveratrol's benefits. There are supplements available in shops and online if you're interested in giving them a try.

Creatine

The natural substance creatine is crucial for the metabolism of energy. It naturally exists in the body, primarily in the muscles and to a lesser extent in the brain. Even though it's a well-liked supplement, some foods—specifically, animal items like meat, fish, and eggs—contain it. Interestingly, those who don't eat meat can benefit from creatine tablets by improving their memory and cognitive function.

Caffeine

The most popular sources of caffeine are dark chocolate, tea, and coffee. Caffeine is a natural stimulant. Taking it as a supplement is an option, but since you can obtain it from these sources, there is no need to.
It works by stimulating your brain and central nervous system, which awakens you and helps you feel less weary.

Studies have proven that caffeine can increase your energy levels and enhance your memory, reaction times, and overall brain function. One cup of coffee typically contains between 50 and 400 mg of caffeine, though this can vary. Single doses of 200–400 mg per day are often seen to be safe and sufficient for health benefits for the majority of persons.

However, consuming too much caffeine can have negative effects, including anxiety, nausea, and difficulty falling asleep.

Phosphatidylserine

Your brain contains phospholipids, a type of fat component that includes phosphatidylserine. Phosphatidylserine supplements have been proposed as a potential aid in maintaining brain health.

According to studies, consuming 100 mg of phosphatidylserine three times a day may help slow the deterioration of brain function that comes with ageing. Additionally, it has been demonstrated that taking phosphatidylserine supplements up to 400 mg daily improves thinking and memory in healthy individuals. But before its impacts on brain function can be fully understood, larger research must be conducted.

Acetyl-L-carnitine
The amino acid acetyl-L-carnitine is created by your body naturally. It is crucial to your metabolism, especially for the creation of energy. It has been asserted that using acetyl-L-carnitine supplements will increase alertness, enhance cognition, and reduce age-related memory loss. You may buy

these supplements online or at vitamin stores. Supplemental acetyl-L-carnitine has been found in several animal experiments to improve learning ability and delay age-related decreases in brain function. Studies on people have revealed that it might be a helpful supplement for halting age-related loss in brain function. Additionally, it might help those with mild dementia or Alzheimer's disease improve their brain function. There is little evidence to support its therapeutic effects on otherwise healthy individuals who are not experiencing a loss of brain function, nevertheless.

CHAPTER 5

BOOSTING YOUR IMMUNE SYSTEM SUPPLEMENTS

Your immune system may be weakened by vitamin deficiencies, including those in zinc, vitamin C, and other nutrients. These vitamins can support immune system function when taken as supplements. A fat-soluble substance called vitamin D is necessary for the well-being and proper operation of your immune system. Monocytes and macrophages, two key components of your immune system's defence, are boosted by vitamin D in their ability to combat pathogens. It also reduces inflammation, which aids in promoting an effective immunological response. This vital vitamin is often lacking in people, which may have a detrimental effect on immune system performance. Upper respiratory tract infections, such as influenza and allergic asthma, are more common in people with low vitamin D levels. According to certain research, taking vitamin D supplements may enhance immune function. Actually, according to the current study, consuming this vitamin may offer protection against respiratory tract infections.

Vitamin D supplementation significantly reduced the incidence of respiratory infections in those with vitamin D deficiency and lowered infection risk in those with adequate vitamin D levels, according to a 2019 analysis of randomised control studies including 11,321 persons.

This hints at a generalising protective effect.

According to other research, vitamin D supplementation may help patients with some illnesses, such as hepatitis C and HIV, respond better to antiviral medications.

For most people, 1,000 to 4,000 IU of additional vitamin D per day, depending on blood levels, is adequate; however, those with more severe deficiencies frequently need considerably larger dosages.

Nutrition D

A lot of research has been done on it about COVID-19 because of how it affects the immune system. According to studies, vitamin D helps quicken recovery and reduce respiratory system irritation. A recent fast-review study concluded that additional studies are required before vitamin D supplements are advised for the prevention and treatment of COVID-19.

However, a lot of experts in the medical and scientific fields contend that taking vitamin D supplements is generally harmless and may even assist people to avoid getting the illness.

Zinc

The element zinc is frequently included in dietary supplements and other healthcare items like lozenges that are designed to strengthen your immune system. This is because zinc is crucial for the health of the immune system. Zinc is essential for immune cell growth and communication, as well as for the inflammatory response. Additionally, zinc specifically safeguards the body's tissue barriers and aids in blocking the entry of external infections.

Your immune system's capacity is greatly impacted by a shortage of this nutrient, which raises your risk of infection and sickness, including pneumonia. A zinc shortage has been proven to be the cause of 16% of all deep respiratory infections worldwide. Around 2 billion individuals worldwide suffer from zinc insufficiency, which is extremely common among senior citizens. This vitamin is thought to be insufficient in up to 30% of older persons.

In affluent nations and North America, zinc deficiency is quite uncommon. However, due to consumption or absorption, many people in the United States have a little zinc shortage. The danger is often higher for older people.

Zinc supplementation may offer protection against respiratory tract infections like the common cold, according to numerous research. Furthermore, those who are already ill may benefit from taking zinc supplements. In a 2019 study, consuming 30 mg of zinc daily reduced the overall duration of the infection and the length of the hospital stay by an average of 2 days compared to a placebo group in 64 hospitalised children with acute lower respiratory tract infections (ALRIs).

A zinc supplement may also shorten the length of a typical cold. Zinc furthermore has antiviral properties. For healthy people, using zinc on a long-term basis is usually safe as long as the daily dose is below the established maximum limit of 40 mg of elemental zinc. Overdosing could prevent copper from being absorbed, which would make you more susceptible to illness.

C vitamin

Given the vital role that vitamin C plays in immune function, vitamin C may be the most widely used supplement for infection prevention. This vitamin helps immune cells operate properly and improves their capacity to fight illness. Additionally, it is required for cellular death, which helps maintain the function of your immune system by removing outdated cells and replacing them with fresh ones.

Additionally, vitamin C serves as a potent antioxidant, preventing damage brought on by oxidative stress, which develops when reactive molecules known as free radicals build up. Stress can impair immune function and is associated with a wide range of illnesses, which could make you more susceptible to infection.

Upper respiratory tract infections, such as the common cold, can be treated more effectively and for a shorter amount of time by taking vitamin C supplements.

Regular vitamin C supplementation at an average dose of 1-2 grammes per day shortened the duration of colds by 8% in adults and 14% in children, according to a major evaluation of 29 trials involving 11,306 persons. Intriguingly, the research also showed that routinely taking vitamin C supplements decreased the likelihood of getting the common cold in people who were under a lot of physical stress, such as marathon runners and soldiers, by up to 50.

Furthermore, it has been demonstrated that high-dose intravenous vitamin C therapy greatly reduces symptoms in patients with severe infections, including sepsis and acute respiratory distress syndrome (ARDS) brought on by viral infections. However, according to other studies, further research is needed to determine the effect of vitamin C in this situation.

Overall, these findings support the notion that immunological function may be greatly impacted by vitamin C supplements, particularly in people whose diets are deficient in the vitamin. The maximum daily dose of vitamin C is 2,000 mg. Daily supplement doses range normally from 250 to 1,000 mg.

Elderberry

Research is being done on the effects of black elderberry (Sambucus nigra), which has traditionally been used to cure illnesses. Elderberry extract exhibits high antibacterial and antiviral potential against bacterial pathogens that cause upper respiratory tract infections and influenza virus strains in test-tube investigations.

Additionally, it has been demonstrated to improve immune system response and may lessen cold duration and severity as well as symptoms connected to viral infections.

Elderberry supplements considerably decreased upper respiratory symptoms brought on by viral infections, according to a study of 4 randomised control studies involving 180 participants.

An older, 5-day research found that those with the flu who took 1 tablespoon (15 mL) of elderberry syrup four times a day saw symptom improvement four days earlier than those who didn't take the syrup and needed fewer prescription drugs. The manufacturer of elderberry syrup financed this old study, which may have tainted the findings. Although elderberry may help with the symptoms of some diseases and the flu virus, we also need to be cautious of the hazards. Some claim that elderberries can increase the production of cytokines to an excessive level, which may harm healthy cells.

For this reason, several experts advise against using elderberry supplements after the early stages of COVID-19.

The usage of elderberry for COVID-19 has not been studied in any published research trials, it should be emphasised. These suggestions are based on earlier studies on elderberries.

According to a holistic assessment of elderberry, various influenza A and B strains were inhibited in studies involving lab animals and humans. Elderberry should only be used under the supervision of a trained healthcare practitioner to reduce the danger of nausea, vomiting, or cyanide toxicity. Elderberry supplements are typically offered for sale as liquids or capsules.

Medicinal mushrooms

Medicinal mushrooms have been used since ancient times to prevent and treat infection and disease. Many types of medicinal mushrooms have been studied for their immune-boosting potential. Over 270 recognized species of medicinal mushrooms are known to have immune-enhancing properties. Cordyceps, lion's mane, maitake, shitake, reishi, and turkey tail are all types that have been shown to benefit immune health. Some research demonstrates that supplementing with specific types of medicinal mushrooms may enhance immune health in several ways as well as reduce symptoms of certain conditions, including asthma and lung infections.

For example, a study in mice with tuberculosis, a serious bacterial disease, found that treatment with cordyceps significantly reduced bacterial load in the lungs, enhanced immune response, and reduced inflammation, compared with a placebo group. In a randomized,

8-week study in 79 adults, supplementing with 1.7 grams of cordyceps mycelium culture extract led to a significant 38% increase in the activity of natural killer (NK) cells, a type of white blood cell that protects against infection.

Turkey tail is another medicinal mushroom that has powerful effects on immune health. Research in humans indicates that turkey tail may enhance immune response, especially in people with certain types of cancer. Many other medicinal mushrooms have been studied for their beneficial effects on immune health as well. Medicinal mushroom products can be found in the form of tinctures, teas, and supplements.

Other supplements with immune-boosting potential

Aside from the items listed above, many supplements may help improve immune response:

• Astragalus. Astragalus is a herb commonly used in traditional Chinese medicine (TCM). Animal research suggests that its extract may significantly improve immune-related responses.

- **Selenium**: Selenium is a mineral that's essential for immune health. Animal research demonstrates that selenium supplements may enhance antiviral defence against influenza strains, including H1N1.

- **Garlic**: Garlic has powerful anti-inflammatory and antiviral properties. It has been shown to enhance immune health by stimulating protective white blood cells like NK cells and macrophages. However, human research is limited.

- **Andrographis**: This herb contains andrographolide, a terpenoid compound found to have antiviral effects against respiratory-disease-causing viruses, including enterovirus D68 and influenza A.

- **Licorice**: Licoricecontains many substances, including glycyrrhizin, that may help protect against viral infections. According to test-tube research, glycyrrhizin exhibits antiviral activity against severe acute respiratory-syndrome–related coronavirus (SARS-CoV).

- **Pelargonium sidoides**: Some human research supports the use of this plant's extract for helping alleviate symptoms of acute viral respiratory infections, including the common cold and bronchitis. Still, results are mixed, and more research is needed.

- **B complex vitamins**: B vitamins, including B12 and B6, are important for a healthy immune response. Yet, many adults are deficient in them, which may negatively affect immune health.

- **Curcumin**: Curcumin is the main active compound in turmeric. It has powerful anti-inflammatory properties, and animal studies indicate that it may help improve immune function.

- **Echinacea:** Echinacea is a genus of plants in the daisy family. Certain species have been shown to improve immune health and may have antiviral effects against several respiratory viruses, including respiratory syncytial virus and rhinoviruses.

- **Propolis**: Propolis is a resin-like material that honeybees produce for use as a sealant in hives. Though it has impressive immune-enhancing effects and may have antiviral properties as well, more human research is needed.

According to results from scientific research, the supplements listed above may offer immune-boosting properties. However, keep in mind that many of the potential effects these supplements have on immune health have not been thoroughly tested in humans, highlighting the need for future studies.

CONCLUSION

"Pill Potency: Harnessing the Potential of Medications for Optimal Health" has taken us on an illuminating voyage into the realm of medicine's remarkable influence on our well-being. Throughout this exploration, we've delved into the concept of Pill Potency – a dynamic force that encompasses the profound impact of medications on our lives. From ancient herbal remedies to cutting-edge pharmaceutical breakthroughs, the evolution of Pill Potency has been a testament to human ingenuity and the ceaseless quest for better health. We've witnessed how medications, carefully developed and administered, can alleviate pain, enhance mood, manage chronic conditions, and even stimulate cognitive function. The pages of this book have been graced with stories of individuals whose lives have been transformed by the remarkable potential of pills.

Yet, it's crucial to acknowledge that Pill Potency is not a standalone solution.

Medications are powerful tools, but their effectiveness is maximized when integrated into a holistic approach to health. We've explored the importance of responsible pill usage, medical supervision, and lifestyle changes that complement the benefits of medications. In our pursuit of well-being, Pill Potency is an essential component, harmonizing with the mind-body connection and the broader context of individual health. As we've journeyed through the categories of Pill Power, from pain relief to immune support, we've also confronted myths and misconceptions, dispelling the notion of pills as magical fixes. Realistic expectations, informed decisions, and open communication with healthcare professionals form the foundation of a successful Pill Power experience.

In closing, "Pill Potency: Harnessing the Potential of Medications for Optimal Health" invites you to recognize and respect the awe-inspiring influence of medications in our lives. It calls upon us to wield Pill Potency responsibly, to integrate it into a broader wellness narrative, and to appreciate its role in shaping a healthier, more vibrant future. The journey of Pill Potency is ongoing, an ever-evolving testament to human dedication, scientific progress, and the remarkable capacity of medicine to enhance and enrich our lives.

9 798886 213882 5